DISCOVER

HEALTH

AND

WELLNESS

DEDICATION

This book is dedicated to the thousands of patients that believe in the Discover Health and Wellness purpose to change the way our world views healthcare. It is because of you that our mission exists. Thank you for putting your trust in our hands. Together we are making a difference. Together we are changing the way our world views healthcare. Together, we are breaking the shackles of medical dependency and introducing a better health care system based on wellness, not sickness. We love you. We thank you. We are here for you.

CONTENTS

INTRODUCTION

WELCOME TO DISCOVER Health and Wellness! In this book, you will find the collaboration of the doctors that have devoted their life mission to helping others discover their true health potential. The pages ahead will explain who they are, why they do what they do, and why it is important to you. The formula for health and wellness exists in five main categories: Toxicity, Nervous System Function, Nutrition, Exercise, and the Health Mindset.

Do you want better health? I think most of us do. Do you want more energy? Do you want to become more vibrant and radiant? Do you just want to get out of pain and no longer be reliant on medication? Discover Health and Wellness will show you how to get there. To get started, read our promise to you . Your healthier, more vibrant, more energetic you, awaits.

THE DISCOVER HEALTH AND WELLNESS PROMISE

1) Our purpose is to change the way our world views healthcare.
2) We serve with an inviting and efficient office. Through personal attention we inspire and build relationships as well as empower through education.
3) Each service we provide is accurate, effective, and of superior quality.
4) With an enthusiastic attitude, we serve with graciousness and commitment to excellence.
5) We instill trust through integrity and compassion.
6) Our approach to healthcare is relevant and progressive. Our office continually strives for controlled efficiency while creating a healing environment.
7) We aggressively provide opportunities for our community to experience a better way of life.
8) As a self-directed team we are passionate and driven. We are committed to leading by example, focusing on results and communicating effectively. The foundation of our team is built on commitment, respect, and loyalty to one another.
9) God's presence and guidance empowers us to be a beacon of light and example for our community.
10) We continually operate in abundance as a result of the value we provide to our community.

CHAPTER 1
THE DHW PURPOSE

LET'S GET STARTED! I have the privilege of starting you off on this journey we call wellness. My name is Dr. Keppen Laszlo and I am the Founder and Clinic Director for Discover Health and Wellness. Our company was born in 1999 and has grown to become one of largest groups of health and wellness centers in our state. As a Palmer Graduate, I have always loved the quote by the Developer of Chiropractic, Dr. BJ Palmer that says, *"You never know how far reaching something you think, say, or do will affect the lives of millions tomorrow."* Discover Health and Wellness, DHW, is leading the wellness way taking those wise words to action.

I became a chiropractor to help people and lead the path for those who have fallen victim to the modern model of healthcare in which we take drugs to cover up symptoms in the body. I am still amazed that we actually call this health care. We are not against the medical system. We are for the medical system when it comes to emergency and sick care. If our patients have tried natural first, then we call our medical friends. The reverse of this order is what has the system in such array. As you will read in the upcoming chapters, the medical first way of healthcare is far from healthy and is extremely deadly and destructive. Are you still taking drugs for healthcare? That era is over.

This chapter is here to show you exactly who Discover Health and Wellness is and why it is important to you.

Discover Health and Wellness' brand is Healthy Healthcare. When patients think of our name, we want them to think of Service, Quality, and Results. Simply put, we give life transforming results through quality care. We are not only the back pain, neck pain, and headache experts. We are the wellness and prevention experts. We specialize in getting patients well through long lasting results utilizing the perfect combination of chiropractic, massage, and toxicity cleanses.

WELLNESS ORIENTATION

I would like to start with a wellness orientation. Now first off, let's take a look at our current healthcare system. This is what most of us are trained to do; we get sick, we go to the medical doctor, we get drugs, than more drugs from the side effects of the first drugs, than surgery. Is this working? The answer is no. I have never met a single person who thought to themselves, "give me more drugs because I want to be healthier." 70% of Americans now take prescription drugs. *Mayo Clinic June 19, 2013*

We are taught to ignore the source of the problem and take the medication. Our body begins to shut down and loose function, and we are taught to take more medication.

The leading causes of preventable death are heart disease, cancer, medical error, respiratory infection, and stroke. Most times, these diseases are preventable. The key to not getting these diseases is to live like you have them now. Limit the medications you are on through your medical doctor, make sure your spinal posture and nervous system are healthy, eat right, exercise, and practice what we call the elevate mindset. We will go into each of these.

It's not an accident that we have more heart disease and cancer than any other country in the world. Of the 787,000 people that died in 2011 of cardiovascular disease, how many of them do you think were on high blood pressure pills and cholesterol lowering drugs? *American Heart Association December 17, 2014.* Would you guess most of them? Heart disease is the number one disease killer and most people I know are on these drugs. I wouldn't call myself a rocket scientist but I don't think taking drugs is preventing heart disease. Do you? If you want to live a long and happy life, we must change the way we look at our health. We must. I care about you, and your kids, and our community and I don't want to see you or your families suffer.

We do have the best system in the world for emergency medicine. We're number one at that, but taking medication for our symptoms instead of addressing the cause of the symptoms is early death, bottom line. Save medicine for sickness and disease and use wellness for health and vitality. Most of us are trained to take medicine from the time we are kids. Have you ever wondered why we all call the metal box with a mirror on it in the bathroom a medicine cabinet? We are trained early.

PREVENTION

My father died of a heart attack at 53 years old. He never met my two boys. He left all of us way too early. Most of our doctors' parents and grandparents suffered from cardiovascular disease and cancer. We see the pain that early death causes to families. My dad died at 53, but was dead much earlier. This is what I mean. Most people don't exercise, have poor lifestyle habits, never took care of their spine, and take medications every time they have symptoms. That lifestyle is early death. It is death before the physical death. The time to address wellness is now. Do you understand that we don't catch heart disease or cancer? We don't catch it. Only 5-10% of cancers are genetic, that's it. The remaining 90-95% of cancers have their roots in the environment and lifestyle. *Pharmaceutical Research. 2008 Sep; 25(9): 2097–2116* .

My colleague had a wealthy patient come in that was 70 years old. He had a walker. If you have been around 70 year olds much, it is easy to see which ones have taken excellent care of themselves and which ones have not. We have had 70 year old patients that still run marathons. This particular gentleman had pain all over his body. He couldn't play with his grand kids. The man was miserable. He told my colleague that he would pay him a million dollars if he could fix him. My colleague looked at his x rays and everything was fused from neglect. There was nothing he could do. He was going to pay him a million dollars. How much is your health worth? Priceless. It is everything.

Here's the challenge, most of us don't take care of our health until we are ready to die. We don't take care of ourselves until we have symptoms-headaches, back pain, chest pain, a chronic cough, etc. When we do get these symptoms, we are trained to cover them up with drugs. Let me ask you, if you were driving down the highway and your oil light came on, would you put a piece of masking tape over the light?

A BETTER APPROACH

There is a better approach. Health comes from how well your body is functioning. It has nothing to do with symptoms. Have you ever heard of the guy who dropped dead from a heart attack and felt great the day before? It happens daily. Did you know that by the time a person is diagnosed with cancer, it has been growing in their body for years? Health has nothing to do with your symptoms. Health is based on function. That is the key. All function starts with your nervous system. God put this amazing healing power in your brain and spinal cord. This is nothing to believe in. If I cut my arm, it doesn't matter if I believe in that power or not, it is going to heal. Your body is a self healing self regulating machine that we are not in control of. You have messages going from your brain down your spine and to all the organs in your entire body. Your nervous system controls absolutely everything in your body. When your spine is lined up properly, your nervous system is flowing at 100% . That's 100% function.

If you want a long, happy, and healthy life, we must take care of our spines. It is everything. It is the structure in which your nervous system flows. This isn't rocket science. If I choke and pinch the nerves that are going to the stomach, what will happen to the stomach over time? The organ will lose function. It doesn't matter if its heartburn, headaches, or epilepsy, we move the bone, get pressure off of the nervous system, and the body heals itself to the best of its ability.

TEST TIME

So it's time for a test. If you are coughing and sneezing, are you sick or healthy? What is your body doing when it is coughing and sneezing? It is working. It is doing what it is supposed to do to get all the bacteria and virus out of you. Symptoms are your friend. Symptoms are the bodies way of saying, "Help me. I am not functioning properly. Don't cover me up with drugs. Fix me." If you have headaches, back pain, neck pain, or asthma for example, your body is saying, "I am not functioning properly and I am sending you pain and symptoms to let you know. I am tensing up the area and decreasing it's function. Get me fixed. My nerves are being chocked and I cannot flow properly to your organs and organ systems." Our most important job is to adjust your spine and turn on your body's healing power to heal itself.

WHO IS DISCOVER HEALTH AND WELLNESS?

Number one, our purpose is to change the way our world views healthcare. Discover Health and Wellness *is* Healthy Healthcare and we achieve that by the following three values:

We find the *source* of your health challenge. We will not cover up your pain, or health challenge with more *medication*. We will find the source of it. We run tests for our patients that can reveal adrenal stress fatigue, chemical toxicity, undetected nerve damage, and much more. Once we find out what is causing the symptoms, we can get to the source of it.

We provide natural health care *first* through corrective care chiropractic, massage, and toxicity cleanses. If referral is necessary, the medical doctors we work with understand that more medication is typically not the answer.

We are a *wellness* center. We believe you are a *whole* person, and we *care* about you as a *whole* person. You are more than a health challenge to us. As a *wellness* center, we show you how to: avoid toxins, eat better, exercise more, think better, and how to have a healthy spine. If you have a health challenge, whether its back pain, neck pain, headaches, fatigue, weight gain, heartburn, asthma, even cancer, if we can help you, we will tell you. If we cannot we will tell you that too.

We are not an office that *only* treats back pain, neck pain, and headaches. We are not an office that treats symptoms and not the causes of the symptoms. And we are not an office that thinks we can cure everything.

WHAT MAKES DISCOVER HEALTH AND WELLNESS REMARKABLE?

There are several things that makes us remarkable, but what really stands out is our wellness approach to health. We have found that all health problems have three main sources: Stress, Toxicity, and Undetected nerve damage.

Most people know that prolonged stress is harmful. Stress is regulated by our adrenal glands. Those glands influence: sleep, digestion, weight gain, allergies, immunity, fatigue, even heart function. We can test your adrenal glands and recommend a protocol that will bring your glands back to normal function eliminating the harmful effects of stress.

There are over 82,000 chemicals that we come into contact with each week. Toxicity leads to weight gain, fatigue, inability to focus, joint pain, and a host of other health problems. We can test your level of toxicity and recommend a specific protocol that will cleanse your body of unwanted toxins improving your overall health, giving you more energy, and help you lose unwanted weight rapidly.

We remove undetected nerve damage. We analyze your spinal curves and get the pressure off of your nervous system by restoring your spinal posture. Undetected nerve damage leads to organ dysfunction, more pain, and eventually a hunched over arthritic posture. Once we get the proper curves back into your spine, you will not only feel so much better, but you will feel years younger.

This specific corrective care wellness approach to health is what really makes us remarkable.

WHAT ELSE MAKES YOU REMARKABLE?

We have been serving the Denver Metro Area since 1999 and our highly educated providers and chiropractors have over 40 years of combined experience. We provide education to elevate your life through quarterly workshops, weekly literature, monthly forums, and online modules. We are incredibly safe. No harmful medications are prescribed to our patients. All of our services are natural. Our offices are medically integrated and our treatments are extremely comfortable, affordable, and based on corrective care objective results with an end date. Our team members and patients volunteer their time and financial resources to many charities every year. We not only help others, we are also environmentally conscious. We are constantly looking for more ways to be green and reduce our imprint. We value the feedback our patients give us. With hundreds of positive testimonials, DHW is thriving, letting us know we are serving our patients well.

WHAT PROBLEMS HAVE YOU SOLVED?

We feel that there are three main problems with our modern model of healthcare today. It's expensive, doesn't work very well, and is dangerous! Patients that seek out Discover Health and Wellness are people who want healthy healthcare, people who are concerned with the rising costs of insurance and need affordable plans, and people who have a health challenge that they are concerned about. DHW is the solution. We have affordable care plans, a better model of healthcare, and are extremely safe.

WHAT ARE THE BENEFITS OF COMING TO DISCOVER HEALTH AND WELLNESS?

Would you like to live your life without your current health challenge? Here's the benefit, live your life without the hassle of poor health or symptoms. Do you want to be pain free? Do you want a leaner body? Do you want more energy and better relationships with your friends and family? Do you want to make more money in your career? Once you finally get the answer to your healthcare challenge and tackle it, your life will elevate. Everything in your life will approve with better health. Discover Health and Wellness is Healthy Healthcare.

DOES DISCOVER HEALTH AND WELLNESS HAVE A GUARANTEE?

DHW absolutely has a guarantee. We have a lot of guarantees. Here is our guarantee to you. You will know exactly what it is going to take to get well in our offices. This will include your care plan and your home exercises. You are a valued patient in our offices. We care about you as a person and as a patient. We only accept patients that we know we can help. As patients ourselves, we expect our doctor to care about our health, so we promise you, as a patient in our offices, we do care about you. If we can help you, we will tell you. If we cannot, we will tell you that too. We will be 100% focused on you and your care. You have entered our offices to get well, and stay well. We take that extremely seriously. Our focus will be on delivering excellent care and service. We will respect your time. Your office visits will have minimal waiting time. We run efficient offices, and we want to help as many people as possible, without compromising the quality of your care. We will answer all of your questions. If we don't know the answer, we will find out by your next visit. We will give you the best care on the planet. We travel the country several times a year learning how to better take care of you. We are here to serve you. We want you to have an excellent experience with everyone and every aspect of our offices. If you are ever dissatisfied with our service, we encourage you to let us know, and we will make it right. This is the DHW guarantee.

WHAT ARE THE TOP QUESTIONS DISCOVER HEALTH AND WELLNESS GETS FROM OUR PATIENTS?

Do adjustments hurt? The answer is NO. In our offices, our adjustments are very comfortable. If a patient has a very tender spot that we need to adjust, we make every effort to make sure it is delivered very effectively without pain.

Is it expensive? Once again the answer is definitely not. Our care is very affordable and if there is any financial concern, we will have a specific plan that will work within your budget.

Do I have to go forever? No. We have specific care plans with an end date. We do encourage patients to receive wellness care at either once or twice a month following correction, however, how long you decide to benefit from a healthy spine and nervous system is always up to you.

Are chiropractors real doctors? Yes! We are real doctors. We have the same four year undergraduate study requirements as medical doctors. We need to get accepted into chiropractic college for another four years of study and then we must get licensed by our state board as Doctors of Chiropractic.

Is chiropractic safe? Yes! Chiropractic care is extremely safe. This is proven by our malpractice premiums being about 1/8 of medical malpractice insurance. Statistically, you have more of a chance getting hit by a falling airplane part, then getting seriously injured from a chiropractor.

CHAPTER ONE CONCLUSION

This chapter now has you well acquainted with who we are, what makes us remarkable, and what the many benefits are to you. Now that you know what Discover Health and Wellness is about, let's dive into what wellness is about.

CHAPTER 2

NUTRITION – EAT YOUR WAY TO WELLNESS OR DISEASE

MY NAME IS Dr. Phillip Wygonski and I have dedicated myself to teaching others how to improve their quality of life. I strive to open people's minds up to a new way of thinking about their health and how chiropractic can help them to get there.

I was born in Cleveland, Ohio. Don't feel bad for me, it was a fun place to grow up. Ohio houses the Rock and Roll of Fame, Cedar Point and the Cleveland Browns. My dad is a carpenter and my mom works accounts receivable. I learned at a young age that things weren't handed to you and that if you wanted something you had to work for it. So growing up I learned my father's trade and became skilled with my hands. As I pursued a career in carpentry, my younger brother who was diagnosed with scoliosis at a young age was getting progressively worse.

My brother Mark being 16 years old didn't want to have another operation. His first two operations were when he was 2 and 4 years old and he was too young to remember them. Now that he was older and understood the risks he thought twice. He did some checking on the internet and discovered that chiropractic can help with scoliosis. My parents made an appointment with the local chiropractor.

The doctor was very nice and answered all my parents questions so they decided to give it a try. My brother started seeing Dr. Hayley regularly. As time progressed x-rays were taken and my brother's scoliosis had stopped progressing and even started to straighten out.

This was a huge win for our family because there were many nights that my parents were stressed about the surgery and the costs and did not know if it would actually fix the problem. Dr. Hayley not only helped my brother and the family, he also made me want to become a chiropractor.

After graduating chiropractic school in 2010, I practiced in one of the largest clinics in Manfield, Ohio for a year and then my love for skiing brought me out to Colorado. Since being out here I have continued to ski every season. I have also learned white water kayaking, downhill mountain biking and hiking. I married my wife, Natalie in Golden, Colorado and we had our son Blake on St. Patricks Day 2015. We enjoy going to all the parks and open spaces, biking and breweries.

Chiropractic in my office is different than most because my goal is to not treat your symptoms but to find the cause of your symptom and correct it.

EATING YOURSELF TO WELLNESS OR DISEASE

Nutrition is a major topic when it comes to health and there are thousands of books and different types of dieting and nutrition plans. It can become overwhelming trying to figure out which one works for you. I remember the first time I tried to lose weight and I started counting calories. I gave up after a day because it was too much work. What I am going to share with you is a simple solution to help you understand why it is important to make good choices with your food in order to express health.

Health is not something you achieve. It is not like a finish line or a dead line you must meet. Health is something your body expresses. When you make poor food choices your body gets sick and when you make good ones you express health.

What do I mean by that? When you set a goal to lose 20 pounds you don't just reach your goal and be done with it. You keep doing those things to keep the weight off and don't go back to your old habits. When you create better and healthier habits you don't develop the problems or health conditions that go along with poor habits. For example, most people look at weight loss/gain as their goal. However weight loss/gain is only the end product of how you eat, exercise, and treat yourself. If you go back to your old ways you will put the weight back on. The other doctors have talked about different aspects of life in order to be healthier and/or happier. What I am going to talk about with you is eating.

WHAT CAN I EAT?

I am not going to tell you what you can or can't have because nobody likes being told what they can't have. But instead, I want to share with you why you should make better food choices and what impact those choices have on your health. Is there anything more important than your health or the health of ones you care about? Stop and think about that. You must have your health to enjoy life. Think back to the last time you were sick. How many friends did you call up or hang out with? Did you get out and do the things you love? How was work when you were sick? Did you call in and stay in bed or sit at your desk and wished you had called off. I know because I have been there.

Even if you're not healthy at this moment, so what! You can change your habits now and you will start to feel better today and your body will function at a higher level. Think of a cigarette smoker. They can smoke a pack a day for years and have all that tar in their lungs. However, if they stop, the body will reverse the damage that was caused and heal the lungs and get rid of the tar.

In order to start a new habit of eating better, first we have to look at your belief system.. One of my mentors Dr. James Chestnut said you're healthy or sick because of the choices you make and those will determine your quality of life. You are in charge of how you exercise, what you think, and what you eat.

As humans we forget that we are animals and that our DNA hasn't changed in thousands of years. We are hunters and gathers. Our bodies were not meant to sit around all day and eat food high in calories with no nutrition and be stressed out of our minds. But yet that is how many people are and they wonder why all these chronic conditions have gone up tremendously. We don't need more drugs and surgery. We need to take care of ourselves. We let ourselves or our kids eat pizza, chips and ice cream. But if our pet tries to eat those things we tell them not to eat that because it is bad for you and you are going to get sick. Yet we don't think twice about eating it. As humans we are animals and our bodies suffer when we eat poor food, don't exercise, and are stressed out.

HEALTH IN A DIFFERENT WAY

Here is an example of health in a different way. Your car has a bunch of different parts that need to work in order for your car to perform, would you agree? Would you agree that how well your car performs is based on the parts in the car. As long as those parts are doing what they are supposed to do your car will get good gas mileage and be reliable. The same goes for the body.

The health of your body is determined by the health of your cells. Any diseases in the body are cells not doing what they should. When your cells are functioning properly you are expressing 100% health. When your body is in a state of stress, which is anything that takes your body away from homeostasis or its normal physiology and decreases cell function. Your cells are either functioning at 100% or they are not. It is that simple. When you are picking your foods, you are either eating something that increases cell function or decreases cell function. Do you think a piece of pizza is moving your cell function up or down? What about an apple? Just like the smokers example I mentioned earlier, you may have eaten salty, greasy foods with loads of preservatives and chemicals in it in the past. However, if you start to make better food choices now, the body can reverse the damage that was done.

I don't have to teach you how to eat because you already know. I want you to understand why you should eat healthy. Good food choices lead to increased cell function. Increased cell function leads to more energy, better mood, less diseases, and a long and better quality of life.

Now I am not telling you that you can never have pizza or your favorite food again. What I want you to do next time you get a craving for something that you know is bad, is to eat one of your favorite fruits or vegetables first. When you eat one of those first the fiber will help fill you up so you do not eat as much pizza. When you start to feel better you will slowly start to eat less food that is bad for you and more that is healthier.

FOOD SELECTION

When picking out your foods try and stay away from the middle of the grocery store because that is where you will find most processed foods. Stick to the outside which will be your fruits, vegetables and meats. When getting fruits and vegetables try and get organic if you can because it contains less chemicals. If you have farmers markets go to those because you can get the fruits and vegetables for less. Choose grass fed organic meat. When the meat is grass fed or raised in its natural environment, it does not have all the inflammation and stress hormones in it.

If you don't take the time to be healthy now then you're going to have to make time when you're sick. Continue to choose the good foods over the bad ones and see health and vitality become your reality.

CHAPTER 3
FITNESS – THE KEYS TO LOOKING GOOD AND FEELING GOOD

HI, I AM Dr. Andrew Hanson. It is my life's passion, my pleasure and my mission to give Denver residents the chiropractic care they need and deserve. I want to share our vision to offer healthy healthcare with the communities of Cherry Creek, Glendale, Aurora and surrounding communities.

Our purpose at DHW is to change the way our world views healthcare. It's my goal to do this every day by educating all of our patients how to properly take care of their spine while dealing with stress and toxicity. Additionally, I hope to inspire my patients to become the best person they can be by staying pain free and keeping the body balanced so that the nervous system can function properly.

I grew up in Pierre, South Dakota where I excelled in football, basketball and tennis. As the quarterback of my high school team, I developed a passion to lead that has remained with me throughout my life. I started my college career in South Dakota where I graduated from a Civil Engineering program. In 2004, I decided to take a risk and move away from my family and friends to attend Colorado State University. At CSU, I received my Bachelors in Sports Medicine and also fell in love with Colorado and the mountains.

After a life changing illness and personal victory in my own health with chiropractic care, I developed a passion for chiropractic and what it had to offer to the world. As a result I have since dedicated my life to sharing the powerful message of chiropractic. In 2008, I attended Parker University in Dallas, Texas. During my time at Parker, I was active in many clubs as well as played on Parker's club tennis team. I graduated from Parker in December of 2011 with my Doctorate of Chiropractic.

Following graduation, I did an internship where I learned from some great chiropractors and furthered my understanding of the miraculous human body. In May of 2013 I joined the wonderful doctors and staff of DHW and in February I opened the beautiful Denver, Colorado location.

I am always expanding my education and knowledge by attending seminars and education classes yearly and if a difficult case comes into the clinic I can consult with one of the several other chiropractors at DHW.

In my free time I enjoy every aspect of Colorado by hiking, trail running, snowboarding, golfing, crossfit training along with a host of other outdoor actives.

I am one of five siblings and I'm very close to my parents, siblings and many nieces and nephews. I welcome you to also join DHW's family of patients. May this year be the year you discover the best version of you.

WHAT IS CHIROPRACTIC?

Chiropractic is a vitalistic philosophy, science, and art which consists solely of the non-therapeutic objective of locating, analyzing, and assisting in the correction of vertebral subluxations, because they are detrimental to the expression of innate intelligence

FITNESS – THE KEY TO LOOKING GOOD AND FEELING GOOD

Have you ever heard the expression "use it or lose it"? It's true! If you don't use your body, you will surely lose it. In this chapter we are going to be talking about the keys to Exercise and more importantly why we need to exercise on a regular basis to not only look good but feel good! The number one reason people exercise is to look good, more bluntly to look sexy, and this is a honorable reason but in most cases we try to set too lofty of goals. Goals to look like celebrities, superheroes or models in the fitness magazines. Now don't get me wrong, I think becoming your best is a great thing but when it comes to looking like a ripped, tanned and 3% body fat model, for most of us it is just not going to happen. Although it may not be attainable for 99% of us, we can still strive to be cut, lean and have a greater self-confidence in how we look and feel.

In today's world there is no shortage of exercise and wellness information. From the internet to world renowned fitness gurus, along with thousands of books and magazines, a person could get overwhelmed real quick. This in itself will lead some to get discouraged and give up because they cannot root out the nonsense and just get to the basics. In this chapter that is just what I am going to do for you. I am going to give you the basics and the motivation in order to begin the process of changing your life. We will first start with top 8 why's you need to exercise and what exercising will do for you. Then we will talk about the 5 best ways to start a program that works for you and keeps you going. In the end you will not only have a place to start but also have a complete on ramp and highway to get you to where you want to be.

WHAT ARE THE TOP 8 BENEFITS OF EXERCISE?

Our purpose at DHW is to change the way the world views health care. My purpose in this chapter is to change the way you view not only exercise but to change why you exercise so it becomes just as important to anything else you do in your life.

To begin with we need to dive into why you need to do some form of exercise and what the top 8 benefits of exercising are. This is in the hopes that you not only exercise to look good but also to feel your best and be your best for yourself, your family and friends. Because let's face it, a lot of people rely on you and when you are not at your best you can't be there for your loved ones.

1) **Exercise Improves Your Posture:** Research is becoming very clear that the better your posture the healthier you are and it has been found that those who exercise have better posture than those that don't. This means that exercise will help with maintaining healthy curves in the spine, increases bone density, and decreases muscle loss. Good posture is important, and one of the best ways to fix your posture is to take care of your spine through adjustments and exercising the muscles in your back. Regularly exercising your abs, back, and other muscles can go a long way into helping your posture, both sitting and standing.

2) **It Reduces Stress And Anxiety:** Anxiety, fearfulness and uncertainty all drain your vitality and dampen your mood, which in turn tends to show on your face and in the way you carry yourself.

Roughly 40 million Americans over 18 suffer from anxiety disorders, according to the National Institutes of Mental Health. *NIMH.*

That's nearly 20 percent of all adults and for many of them, that anxiety strips both the smile from their face and the spring from their step. Exercise has been shown to alleviate most mild to moderate cases of anxiety, and can very quickly improve mood.

Jack Raglin, PhD, a sport psychologist at Indiana University in Bloomington, Ind., is only half-joking when he says, "Exercise is like taking a tranquilizer, but better because you get the side effect of improved health and fitness." Studies out of Raglin's lab suggest that as little as 15 minutes of exercise bestows a calm that can last for hours. As for what kind of exercise elicits the biggest response, he recommends either heart-thumping aerobic exercise, like running, cycling or swimming, or a mixture of aerobic and anaerobic exercise, such as weight training.

3) **You'll Improve Your Memory:** Ever feel like you think a bit more clearly after a good workout? Not only is your brain getting more energy and oxygen, but many studies have shown that exercise can boost your memory and help you learn better. Of course, an intense workout right before a big exam could leave you more tired than smart but the two are still undoubtedly linked.

4) **Greater Self Confidence:** Obviously, exercise can improve your appearance which can improve confidence, but there's more to it than that. Exercise can also help you feel more accomplished and social. Even if you don't see immediate results in your body, that effort will make you feel better and a bit of confidence can go a long way. Confident people radiate a certain physical appeal and charisma. A recent British study found that people who began a regular exercise program at their local gym felt better about their self-worth, their physical condition and their overall health compared with their peers who stayed home. The best part was that their self-worth crept up right away even before they saw a significant change in their bodies.

"You don't need to improve your fitness level to improve your self-perception of how fit you are," says Adrian Taylor, PhD, an exercise researcher at the University of Exeter in England and the study's lead investigator. And from there it's only a short leap to enjoying healthier self-esteem, he adds. "Our self-worth is directly tied to our energy levels, our feelings of competence and our perceived attractiveness." *www.doh.gov.uk* And nothing is more gorgeous than the self-assurance that comes from feeling good in your own skin.

5) **5) More Restful Sleep:** Plagued by dark circles? You're not alone. As many as 60 million Americans wrestle with insomnia, according to a recent Harvard Medical School report. A slew of studies show exercise can elicit longer, more restful sleep. Why? Well, an intense workout may leave you too hungry for shuteye recovery time. But there's more to it than that. Shawn Talbott, PhD, nutritional biochemist and author of The Metabolic Method (*Current Book, 2008*), explains that exercise sharpens the body's sensitivity to the stress hormone cortisol, which can enhance sleep. Sleeping better leaves you looking fresh and healthy.

6) **Have More Energy:** It may seem counter-intuitive after all, working out can drain your energy quite a bit—but regular exercise can actually make you feel more energized throughout the day. In fact, one study found that exercising in the middle of the day can leave you feeling more energetic and productive for the rest of the afternoon. You should still try to get in some walking throughout the day, but a midday workout could be a great pick-me-up.

7) **Get Sick Less Often:** Nobody likes getting sick and exercise can help. A recent study found that people who exercised regularly were half as likely to get a cold, than people who didn't. Exercise's immune-enhancing powers are nothing to sneeze at. Exercise shores up the immune system by stimulating the body into churning out more white blood cells, including neutrophils and natural killer cells. More white blood cells mean fewer bacteria and viruses sneak past the gate. Net effect: You don't get that worn-down sick look that comes from feeling under the weather, and small blemishes and wounds of all kinds heal faster. Exercise also keeps the lymph system happy. The body has roughly 500 lymph nodes, little nodules of tissue that take out metabolic trash. But the nodes can't haul garbage to the curb without the help of nearby muscles. When muscles contract during exercise, they put the squeeze on lymph nodes, helping them pump waste out of your system. Increased circulation is the key to both white blood cell production and better lymph drainage, and the best way to achieve it is to regularly do things that make you breathe harder. That increased blood flow is what revs up the immune system and research shows that just 45 minutes of walking each day can cut the number of days of work you miss because of illness by up to 50 percent.

The takeaway message is simple: there is no supplement or medication that has proven to be as strong as regular exercise in improving the immune system's ability to detect and destroy invaders.

BONUS: You Will Just Be Happier: All these put together equals a much happier you. It's not just those "runner's high" endorphins, regular exercise can actually improve your life in many ways. All you need to do is make it a habit—the University of Bristol found that people's mood significantly improved on days they exercised, so find a way to fit a quick workout into your daily routine and you'll be well on your way.

TOP 5 WAYS TO START EXERCISING

Alright now that we know the top benefits to why you need to exercise and how it can affect every aspect of your life. Let's get into the top 5 ways to start exercising so you can look and feel your best.

1) **Know Just How in Shape You Are:** You need a starting point of where you are at today and then goals to where you want to be in the future. You probably have some idea of what kind of physical shape you're in. But in order to find out where you're truly at you'll need to record your baseline fitness scores. To do this you will want to take these 5 metrics. You can always do more but this will give you good metrics to come back to see just how far you have come. This is also a great time to speak with your doctor and let them know you are starting an exercise program.

    i. Your pulse rate before and after you walk 1 mile (1.6 kilometers)

    ii. How long it takes you to walk 1 mile (1.6 kilometers)

    iii. How many push-ups you can do at a time

    iv. How far you can reach forward while seated on the floor with your legs in front of you

    v. Your waist circumference as measured around your bare abdomen just above your hipbone.

2) **Choose a Goal:** This can be different for each person. Maybe you want to get buff, maybe you want to lose weight, or maybe you just want to fight off heart disease and diabetes. Whatever it is, it'll help you to have a clear goal in mind. With a clear goal, you can stick to it and know if you're on the right path.

Think about what you want to be good at. Maybe you don't have a weight goal or a waistline goal, but you want to be able to run a 5k, no problem. What's more, if you have the desire to be good at it, you'll probably enjoy it. Which we will come back to. That's the key to staying with it.

With this methodology, your goal will be in your workout. Aim for something specific: a 5k in 30 minutes or 30 push-ups a minute, for example. This will be what you're working toward.

Think about what you want to be. Do you want to be 4 inches thinner around the waist? 15lbs lighter? Lose 5% of your body fat? If it's easier for you, think in numbers.

If your goal is weight loss, know that 1kg (2.2 pounds) is 3,500 calories. You need to burn 500 calories a day working out (if you're on a balanced diet) to lose one pound a week.

3) **Choose a Balanced Routine:** If you're looking to be fit overall, you'll want to start a routine that keeps you on top of every aspect of your game that means aerobic exercise, strength training, and flexibility training. All three of them:

Cardiovascular activity: Start out simple with walking or running. Do this for half an hour, five times a week. Try to stay on a level where you could carry a basic conversation, but definitely couldn't carry a tune.

Strength conditioning: Start doing 4 to 8 different exercises, making sure to work out different muscle groups. And don't go for weight—it's better to lift lighter and maintain the right form. Though cardio can and should be done 5 times a week, keep the weight training to twice. Your body needs time to repair itself, quite literally.

Flexibility training: You'll be surprised how much improving your flexibility can help you across the board. Yoga is a great way to improve flexibility and mobility.

4) **Pick a time that can become a habit:** In order to integrate this into your lifestyle, you'll need to make it a priority. To do this, set aside a time at least a few days a week. Whether it's 6:00am or 6:00pm, write it down in pen. There's no getting around it.

Getting over the initial hump will be the hardest part. Soon enough, when 6:00am rolls around, your body will be raring to go and feeling antsy to get that endorphin rush.

5) **Do the Thing You Love:** Some fitness people like to talk tough. They'll say things like "pain is weakness leaving the body" or "if you're enjoying yourself, you're not training." I get where they're coming from because hitting the truly elite levels of performance does require enduring pain and sacrifice and unpleasantness and, frankly, momentary bouts of misery. But even the triathletes subjecting themselves to crippling pain do so out of love. There's some hate there, too, but love is the foundation.

The biggest benefit to doing something you love for exercise is that you'll actually do it. Since the most effective and beneficial exercise is the one you can stick with, this is one way to ensure you obtain the benefits. Do what you love. You'll actually do it and it'll probably give you better results.

FEEL SEXIER

Savor how exercise makes you feel. Good workouts reveal the extremes of subjective human experience. We get butterflies before a big lift or a particularly grueling sprint and feel the real anxiety of knowing you're about to push your body to its limit. We know the joy of victory (even if it's against your last workout) and the crushing dejection of defeat. The ups, the downs and the all-arounds. You're confident after a workout. "Yeah, I just lifted that." You feel sexier, too, because you've proven to yourself and the world that you know how to use and inhabit your body.

Know these feelings. Savor them. They may not be "fun" or "pleasant," but that's not the point. They're proof that you're still alive and that these workouts are doing something.

If you use these strategies you will have the motivation and desire to develop a workout routine that fits you. One that you love and will stick to even when you are feeling that "I don't want to work out feeling." Once you start to feel the benefits of exercise you will always make the time to put the hard work in because you know you are on your way to looking good and feeling good. I am with you on this mission and here to help you reach your goals in this process of rejuvenating your health and wellness.

CHAPTER 4
MINDSET – THE WAY OF THE WELLNESS WARRIOR

MY NAME IS Dr. Dale Zagiba, DC. I am the chiropractor at Discover Health and Wellness Ken Caryl. I attended East Carolina University where I graduated Magna Cum Laude with a B.S. in Exercise Physiology before I pursued my Doctorate of Chiropractic from Palmer College of Chiropractic Florida. I am married to my beautiful wife Lindsie and we have the most amazing son Anthony. I have a passion for helping people find answers to their health issues, by offering natural and safe solutions. Outside of work I love spending time with friends and family, playing sports, exploring the outdoors, and I am a motorcycle enthusiast.

I began a fascination with the spine at an early age. My uncle became a quadriplegic by a pool diving accident. I used to say "I am going to fix your neck!", as I got older I began to pursue a career in medicine. However, things took a turn I never expected. I lost my mom to a brain aneurysm when I was 20 years old and realized that I did not want to be the neurosurgeon in that situation. I wanted to be in a position where I could help people not only with care but with education to live healthier. With some strong guidance by my father I found chiropractic. As soon as I got to chiropractic school I knew this was my calling. I get to help people solve their health issues by addressing their cause while improving overall nervous system function and overall health education. I cannot imagine doing anything else for a living; I love waking up and taking care of patients just like I would my own family every day.

Chiropractic is the removal of nerve interference through spinal alignment. By removing the nerve interference caused by spinal misalignments leads to: improved nerve function, increased joint mobility, prevention of joint and disc disease, increased immune system, and much more. When we improve the health of our spine and nervous system it affects everything, thus improving our quality and quantity of life.

MINDSET OF A WELLNESS WARRIOR

As the famous quote goes, "Worrying is like a rocking chair. It gives you something to do but it doesn't get you anywhere." The mindset of a wellness warrior is truly a simple one, yet as simple as it is accomplishing this mental state, it is much more challenging and takes work to achieve and years to master. Just ask any of the Doctors at Discover Health and Wellness. At Discover Health and Wellness we all know we are works in progress, but we know deep inside that we are all amazing, capable, loving, and passionate people out there working to improve the wellness and health of our patients, our communities, and ourselves. This is my opportunity to spread my knowledge and experience to show each and every one of you how your mindset is key to becoming a wellness warrior.

I was born lucky enough to have parents that instilled a belief in me that I could be anything as long as I put my mind to it. I'm actually pretty sure that is exactly how they said it. Put your mind to it. As I have progressed in life I have learned how valuable those words really are to me, but it is not the words, it is how the words turned into a mindset that sets me up for life. The concept that when I wake up every morning I know today is going to be amazing, good things will happen, and I will grow as a person today. Now mindset is not the only thing you need, it would sure be nice that if I believed I was going to have someone hand me a million dollars today that would be all that I need to do for it to come to fruition. Sorry to break it to you guys, but that is just not the way the world works. You have to take action on your goals/dreams to make them a reality.

My mindset is the juice that helps me put my ideas to action, and my actions take me closer and closer my dreams. Without the right mindset it will be much more difficult to keep your stance when you are taking hits from your challenges, or to keep up the courage to take action when nerves and fear kick in. Another issue that arises is maybe you might be taking action but you have the mindset that you are not getting anywhere. Have you heard the saying "mind over matter"? There is a lot of truth to it and it can work in both ways, either for your benefit or your own downfall. The thing is most people don't even realize that it is their own beliefs and mental state that can cause this problem. Most people have a great attitude 90% of the time, then difficulties, challenges, even life altering events come up, and this is where your mental toughness and mindset either kicks in and elevates you to greatness, or it fizzes out and so do you, your dreams, and your goals. So, what is it going to be? Are you going to be an excuse ridden-postponing-procrastinator? Or are you going to be a no excuses, get it done, fall 9 times get up 10 champion?. Mindset is what will determine your answer, so whatever it is in your life start today. Put simply, change your mindset and change your life.

WHAT DO YOU WANT?

What do you want? Really, think about this for a second. Do you know what you want? Do you have goals? Do you know where you want to be in 5, 10, 30 years from today? Knowing what you want or where you want to be is crucial to have the right mindset, but more importantly it helps you keep the motivation necessary to take action on what you need to do. One of the biggest mistakes people make is they don't make smart goals, people make vague ones "I want to lose weight this year", "I want to start saving this year", "I'm going to start exercising more". Listen these are all great things however, they leave a lot of ambiguity. There are no guidelines in place and in fact there is no real goal in place just general thoughts. For example, saying I want to lose weight is not a good goal. I want to lose 30 pounds in 6 months is. We have given a specific result that we can track and that is what is needed. This way we can see how far we have come or how much work is left to do. This is huge. That way when our time frame is up if we didn't hit our mark is it time to give up and move on? Heck no, it is time to readjust and keep going after it. One of the biggest problems people make is that as soon as they make the first slip up on their goal they basically call it quits. Folks we should all know by now quitters never win, but that is what happens to a lot of people. "Guess, I'll have to do better next year." No! Do not be in agreement with this. Try this instead, "well I made it this far, but I had some challenges and I didn't make my goal. Let's push it out another 6 months and I know I will hit it this time." That is the mindset of a warrior that gets where they want to go. Another benefit of being crystal clear on what you want is that it will give you motivation to keep pushing when challenges pop up. When your end result is on your mind it is easier to make the small sacrifice now, versus giving in and suffering the ultimate sacrifice of giving up your goals. It's easy to say, hey I deserve that donut, I am too tired to exercise today, STOP right now think about what kind of pain that will cause in the end and then make the right choice. This is simple but far from easy.

You have to attach major pain to making the small choices we make. If I don't do my exercises today, I will get off track, if I get off track I will be in more pain and may need surgery. Seem intense? Good because I want it to. Same thing though with the other side because sometimes pain scares people into doing nothing. Let's try it the other way with massive pleasure on making the slightly harder better choice. If I do my exercises my spine will be corrected, which means I won't be in pain, I won't need surgery, and I will be able to play with my grandkids any way they want. Works just as well, but the thing is the focus is on the end result not the choice you're making right now.

WHY AM I DOING THIS?

The next thing a wellness warrior is crystal clear on is why they are doing what they are doing. Knowing what you want is crucial with that said, it is just as vital to know why you want what you want or why your purpose is so important to you. Without a strong why it makes it much more difficult to make the hard choices when they arise. When your why or purpose is crystal clear it gives you strength and insight to make the hard choices when they arise. There is an understanding deep inside that the pain of making the hard choice is far less than the pain of making the easy choice now because it will either pay in dividends years down the road or your consequences will be compounded.

For example, when a lot of patients come into our offices they think they are there because they have back pain, neck pain, headaches, or some kind of physical problem. The truth is they are coming to us because deep inside of them they have a deeper reason they just might not be aware of yet. People come to our office because they want to feel well, they want to have good health, they want to make sure they can keep working, they want to be able to play on the floor with their grand-kids, they want to live long enough to knock things off their bucket list, and this could go on. The point is generally people always have a deeper reason for making the choice we make, but when we know what we want and why we want it gives us motivation to make the hard choices that take us where we want to go in the long run rather than the easy way out which will give us the temporary pleasure that hinders our long term goals and desires. These are the kind of questions the wellness warrior is thinking about before making every choice they make. Find out your deeper why, and tap that into your mindset to give yourself a constant and consistent source of motivation to keep your head in the game and accomplish your goals.

NO EXCUSES

Excuses are a one way trip to self-victimization and it is no place for any warrior of any kind. Bad things happen, sometimes really bad things happen. Even worse they happen out of our realm of direct control. This is life friends however, when we believe that things are out of control it can lead to a slippery slope of feeling powerless. One excuse usually leads to another and another and another, and next thing you know you have washed yourself clean of everything in your life, your fault or not. Now you have become a helpless victim and are at the mercy of your environment. This is a scary place to be. When people end up in this place of no control there is no fight, no battle, just sitting there taking punch after punch just hoping you will survive the next hit.

Sounds pretty terrible right? Well what can I do you might ask? The first thing to do is to start taking full responsibility today and not let your challenges make you a powerless victim. If something is out of your control you can get control simply, but not easily. The answer is to take responsibility for everything in your life even if those things could not be prevented. For example one of the biggest excuses I hear is "well it is my genetics", "I can't help it I was born this way". REALLY? Are you are going to leave something that is bothering you that way? Oh well, just cope with it till I can't any longer, not the wellness warrior. How about this approach instead, "well I know I have this going against me but I can do X Y and Z to help stop it." Doesn't that sound so much more empowering?

When we take responsibility for things that are out of our control we gain control. The focus is on what we can do about a challenge instead of what this challenge has done to us. The belief is this, "I am not going to let anything define who I am but myself and the choices I make, not the ones that were made for me". Generally there is almost always something you can do about a problem or challenge, as long as you have the right mindset to recognize self-defeating thoughts or excuses to take a proactive role in your health and more importantly your life.

POTENTIAL

What I have wanted you to realize is that we all have the potential to accomplish anything, when the mindset of the warrior has been applied. Life is not there to beat us down, it is there to be enjoyed with the feeling of being young, vital, and full of energy around the people we love and care about. Now obviously my focus is on health and wellness because it is our greatest asset and affects every area of our life, but this can be applied to any challenge or aspect of life. If you have the mindset of a winner or warrior, it is not if but when you will win. We all have lost battles from time to time and that is ok, as long as we learn and grow from them. It is when we keep making the same mistakes over and over and make no changes, only excuses, that we lose. So, whatever your challenge is: your health, your career, your relationships, or whatever it is for you, adapt the mindset of the wellness warrior and get your health in order and take responsibility for your life and like my mentor always says, "Go for it like a starving pit bull goes after a T-bone steak."

CHAPTER 5
NERVOUS SYSTEM FUNCTION – THE MASTER CONTROL CENTER

THIS CHAPTER IS going to tell you about the most important part of your body! The Nervous System. Allow myself to introduce myself. I am Dr. Cameron A. Hall D.C. I am a chiropractor. I never knew how rewarding life could be until I found this profession. Every day I have the opportunity to help someone increase the quality of their life, and the lives of their family. People come in my office with significant health issues and without drugs or surgery they leave my care healthier, more educated, a higher quality of life, less chance of degenerative conditions, and of course pain free. I may be the only person I know that goes in early, stays late, and will even come in on the weekends. The word "doctor" means teacher. Not coverer-upper of symptoms, but teacher. A doctor's real duty is to educate their patients on how to live a healthier life. Treating symptoms is only one aspect of this job. Often-times a patient's symptoms are only the tip of the iceberg, so just working to cover them up is a huge disservice to the patient. A true doctor must not only be able to alleviate a patient's symptoms but also correct the underlying cause of those symptoms. Covering pain up with pain killers is the absolute worst thing you can do. We'll get more in to how to properly deal with symptoms later in this chapter. First, patients are always asking me, "How did you get in to chiropractic?" The best answer on how someone becomes a chiropractor is opportunity. The opportunity presents itself, not unlike fate. I always liked helping people, and I knew I wanted to be in a field where I could make a difference in people's lives. There is no profession that gives you the ability to help in such a profound way other than chiropractic. So when the opportunity presented itself for me to become a chiropractor I jumped on it. This journey has completely changed the way I view life and the world. Even during my first years in grad school I had no idea just how far this profession would take me. What a ride.

THE UNIQUENESS

During grad school, the main concern is diagnosis, diagnosis, diagnosis. We are taught to identify nearly every musculoskeletal condition known to man. During our four year doctorate degree, a full two years of continuous anatomical training and direct hands on training with cadaveric specimens is included to ensure that chiropractors have the best musculoskeletal education in the world. Lucky for our patients we are also taught how to treat them. I mean, you won't be in practice very long if you can't get a patient out of pain. Once I graduated I thought that was going to be my job. A patient comes in with back pain, I diagnose the cause, fix it, and then discharge. Very quickly I found out it wasn't that simple. The patient's pain would go away but more often than not it would come back. Something was missing. I knew I had to find a new model of treatment. Physical Therapists deal mainly with the muscles, and they seem to get some pretty good results. Chiropractors deal mainly with the skeletal system and the spine, and they seem to get pretty good results. So I started looking for something new. I started to learn that you can't just move the bones and not address the muscles. In that same fashion you can't train the muscles without addressing the joint and boney misalignments. What if there was a way to combine both? That is when I found DHW. These doctors were doing things I had never heard of. They had developed a treatment protocol that combines the best areas of both chiropractic and physical rehabilitation. They were actually fixing patients' spines, not just dealing with their pain. I was blown away. Not only did they fix patients' spines and completely eliminate their pain, but they also focused on educating the patient on how to live better lives. Again I was blown away. The embodiment of the word 'Doctor', to teach the patient how to live a healthier and high quality of life was here. It was a totally new way of thinking and practicing. They addressed both the bones and the muscles, but also they focused on the nervous system.

THE NERVOUS SYSTEM

The nervous system is what this chapter is all about. Chiropractic was founded on the doctors ability to directly affect the nervous system. Through the years however; the profession has lost much of that original purpose. It was here while rediscovering chiropractic's roots that I learned just how awesome the human body is, and the amazing things that can be done by directly affecting the nervous system. The human body is a wonderful machine, perfectly designed to last us our entire life if it is maintained properly. Behind it all is the body's nervous system. Like the electrical system and computer control centers in your car, your nervous system runs every function of your body; from wiggling your pinky toe to batting your eyes, your nervous system controls everything you do. The nerves themselves can be quite fragile however. Take for example; if you fall asleep on your arm what happens? It falls 'asleep' right? It goes numb. The reason for that is when pressure is applied to the nerves that go into your arm they start to decrease the signals being transmitted. Apply that pressure long enough and boom, your arm goes numb. Now imagine you put the same amount of small pressure on the nerves that go to your heart, or liver. What happens? The exact same loss of signal will happen to any nerve that has pressure applied to it. The problem comes when pressure is applied to nerves that don't have the sensory feed-back loop. What is a sensory feed-back loop you may ask? The nerves in your arms and hands are specialty nerves. They are fine tuned to sense feeling, like touch or vibration. So when pressure is placed on those nerves you get the numb feeling. The nerves that go to your heart, lungs, and liver don't have those types of fibers. So when pressure is placed on those nerves you don't have the same effect as a numb arm, but the organ can still be affected. Make sense?

WHAT IS PAIN?

So how do you know if you have pressure on those types of nerves? Even though you can't feel if the nerves to your heart have pressure on them, what you can feel are the misaligned structures that are putting the pressure. For instance, neck pain and upper back pain aren't just localized issues. They are only a symptom of a much larger issue. Think of pain as a check engine light on your car. The light coming on isn't the problem. The problem is in the engine. You have to pop the hood and take a look. What you will find is a structural issue that has caused pain receptors called 'nociceptors' to activate. That is all pain is, it is a simple receptor that is either, put under too much load, stretched too far or activated. The pain just tells you something is wrong with that area. That is why just dealing with the pain is so dangerous. Putting a piece of tape over your check engine light doesn't fix the problem under the engine. You may not see the light any more but the problem is still occurring in the engine and will get worse until something breaks down. Taking a pain pill for aches and pains is the same thing. You will feel better in the short term but long term you are doing more damage to your body. Deal with what is causing the pain and you will be doing your body a big favor. So let's use neck pain as our example. Everyone has or has had neck pain right? Where neck pain may be one of the most commonly reported alignments in doctor's offices the causes are all relatively the same. Barring, of course, falling down stairs or car accidents, most cases of neck pain start small and progress over the course of an individual's life.

BOWLING BALL

You have to remember you have a ten pound bowling ball sitting on seven small bones and the equivalent of a t-bone steak's worth of muscles to hold up the whole thing. Your cervical spine, neck bones, are specifically designed to hold this bowling ball over a perfect center of gravity. They are actually shaped in a very intricate formation that accomplished this task! Isn't that amazing! Problem is they are made to be in a certain formation and they are also supposed to be used by a bipedal, up right walking, animal, us. So when we sit at our desk for eight hours a day with our heads shifted forward, then we spend our hour lunch looking down at our phone, and then we get home and relax on the couch with a slouchy posture. Long story short, we are not using our body as it was intended. Through all of this the structure of your cervical spine starts to shift forward, and the weight is no longer supported on the bones. The weight is shifted then to the muscles. It is these muscles that will later start to turn on those pain receptors and once they reach a point they can no longer comfortably hold that bowling ball. Through the years people will take pain killers, see a massage therapist, buy an at home neck massager and even seek chiropractic help. The pain remember is just a receptor that has been activated because of something else. Now the neck pain itself is annoying but let's look at what turns the receptors on.

THE SILENT KILLER

Your cervical spine, neck, is the most important structure in your entire body. The cervical spine contains your brain stem and the nerves that control all of your vital functions: heart and lungs just to name a few. So once you start to see those pain signals turn on that means several of your body's automatic compensation mechanisms have failed. Your body is incredibly intelligent and can compensate for these issues up to a point. Once the pain has started, those compensations are starting to fail. Look at these compensations like engineers would look at a dam. When a dam starts to fail the engineers try to reinforce the dam right? Your body will do the same thing. Your body can compensate by activating certain accessory muscles to help "hold" or support the extra load once the bowling ball, head, has shifted forward. It is often these accessory muscles that start to activate those pain receptors later in life, because they were not made to hold that amount of load for that period of time and eventually start to fatigue and get achy. Make sense? Once those receptors have activated the issue has been there for several years. This is where the pain comes from, but what about the nerves? Remember this chapter is about the nervous system? So those bones that we talked about, the fabulous seven, they are specifically designed and shaped so that they can support the weight of a ten pound object for ten hours a day without ever wearing out. They are also shaped so that your spinal canal, the hole that goes through the middle of each bone, line up correctly. But, they have to be in that curved formation. Once your head has shifted forward the bones don't line up correctly. This is what doctor's call "loss of cervical lordosis". It's a fancy word for loss of cervical curve. Once those bones don't line up, neither then does the central canal, and pressure begins to be placed on those all-important nerves and brainstem. This is what we term the silent killer. You'll never feel this pressure, though it is slowly killing you. In a research article published in a medical journal, it was shown that a loss of cervical lordosis can take up to fourteen years off an individual's life span! *Spine, Nov. 1, 2005 Vol. 30 (21) pg. 2388-2392*. Once this pressure is placed on those nerves they start to slowly lose communication with whatever they go to. Unfortunately the nerves in your neck go to your heart and lung primarily. And remind me again what the top two killers of the elderly are? Heart and lung pathology? Yes.

STRUCTURE

Like any machine the human body can show wear and tear if it is not properly maintained. This wear and tear is what we call arthritis. Many people think that arthritis is genetic and unavoidable, but that is simply not the case. Your body's structure is built for two purposes: protection of vital systems and weight distribution. When your structures are not aligned properly then the weight distribution will be altered. Once altered this "weight shift" will start to put more load on certain structure's causing them to wear and tear prematurely. This is what causes arthritic joints. If these structural issues are caught soon enough and correctly, that wear and tear can be prevented. If the joint is already showing degeneration then it can still be halted and prevented from progressing, if the structural issue can be corrected. So how do you know if these issues are going on in your own body? See a chiropractor! Chiropractors are in a unique position to identify and correct these issues. The key word is correct. A lot of patients get caught in what I call the chiropractic cycle. This happens when a patient with neck pain, low back pain, or headaches goes into a chiropractor, they get an adjustment, and their pain feels better. However, a single adjustment is just like an over the counter pain killer. It is only temporary. As we know from reading above the pain is only a symptom of a much larger problem. So by resetting the structure temporarily with a single adjustment then the pain will go away as long as that adjustment holds. As soon as the structure is pulled back out to the altered position the pain comes back and the patient is back in the chiropractor's office. Correcting the structural patterns is the only way to completely eliminate the symptoms and prevent the wear and tear on the structures. To correct the structure it's not just the adjustment. The adjustment is the foundation, by resetting the structure with a chiropractic adjustment you are training a new structure, but that new structure must be reinforced with a new muscle memory. The only way to get the new structure to remain is to train the specific muscle groups responsible for holding that new structure. Once the new pattern starts to form all you have to do is reinforce it. The sign of a great chiropractor is that he or she has a plan for your condition. They should know how long it will take and how many office visits you will need. Correction takes time and it's not an overnight process. The training of the new structure must be structured appropriately. It's starts with the adjustment and ends with the muscle training.

DIAGNOSTIC TESTING

Let's not forget X-rays. Radiographs allow chiropractors to properly diagnose patient's specific issues and they also help to rule out other more serious causes that could be worsened by chiropractic care. Going in to a chiropractor for low back pain could absolutely save your life if one of these more serious issues are identified. You must know what the structure looks like in order to create an effective care plan. Once the chiropractor has laid out your treatment plan and you have completed the protocol then the real test is a new X-ray. If the new structure is holding it will show on the X-ray.

The structural correction is what you can see, what you feel is completely different. Your symptoms are gone which is great, but the real magic is what this does for your nervous system. Once the structure is corrected the pressure being applied to your nerves is eliminated. This is where you hear about the miracles of chiropractic. As a chiropractor I set out to fix your structure. By doing that, yes your pain and symptoms go away, but often times we see truly amazing side effects after care. Patients with depression, irritable bowel syndrome, high blood pressure, heart arrhythmias, gastric reflux, seizures, and so many other conditions have gotten relief. Chiropractic is not a cure-all, there are no such things, and some patients don't see relief in their symptoms. However, if you have neck pain, back pain, headaches, anything, and you haven't tried chiropractic; then please try it. Even if you have tried chiropractic in the past look up one of our centers or a clinic that does structural corrective care and at least see if they can help. You might be surprised.

CHAPTER 6
CHILDREN – THE WELLNESS PATH

MY NAME IS Dr. Branden Teets, DC. I was born and raised in southwestern Pennsylvania and spent my childhood and teenage years in Uniontown and Uledi. After getting my undergraduate degree in biology from Saint Vincent College in Latrobe, PA, I left for Marietta, GA to attend Life University to get my doctor of chiropractic degree. I spent eight months after graduation practicing in Glen Rock, PA under the tutelage of Dr. Karen Barclay, DC. Ultimately, in May of 2011, my family and I packed up and left the comforts of Pennsylvania to move to Aurora, CO to start with Discover Health and Wellness.

One thing people that know me understand is that I love sports. I love to watch them and play them. I won numerous all-star awards in basketball and baseball throughout my teen years, as well as cross country and track. An honor I received my senior year of high school was being voted Most Athletic by my peers and even receiving the Marine Corps Outstanding Athlete award. Now being in my 30's, I focus all of my attention on the love that I just can't quit because I truly love it: running. My current goal is to qualify for the Boston Marathon after years of 5ks and 8ks in high school and college. At the moment my oldest son is quite interested in running since he sees how much it means to his dad.

Running – well, more specifically cross-country is what ultimately called me to becoming a chiropractor. In September of my junior year of high school we were doing our infamous "mile repeat" workout, where we would run a mile on our campus's course and race pace anywhere from 3 to 5 times with rest in between.

On our course, we have a massive incline dubbed "Hell Hill." It is called that for a reason. And during the 2nd repeat that day, while running up Hell Hill, the lower left side of my back seized up and immediately dropped me to all fours. After the intense pain became more manageable, I walked to the top and let my coach know I couldn't continue. A teammate told me that if I wanted to get better, I needed to see his dad. His dad was a chiropractor. Quite honestly, I had never even heard that word before, and I didn't care. I just wanted to run and be with my team.

I went to see Dr. Jodon to get examined and then start care. It didn't take long for my back to release and all pain was gone. In fact, that happened within the first 2 weeks. However, that wasn't the turning point for me. You see, since birth and up until that point, I always had a digestive issue to where I would only have a bowel movement once every week, sometimes every two weeks. That is not normal, and it's dangerous, which is why I was sick a lot as a kid. After roughly 5-6 weeks under Dr. Jodon's care, I was having bowel movements every other day, which to me was not normal. That entire time I was under his care, he had no idea this had plagued me for almost 17 years because I never told him. I was only focused on my back. He sat down with me and taught me what chiropractic was.

I ask my patients this question: what part of your body would you be ok with NOT working at 100% of its functional ability? The answer is always "no part." The only way you can have 100% function within the body is to have proper nerve function and proper never flow from the brain to the body. A subluxation is when a bone or series of bones misalign to put direct pressure on the nerve and/or the spinal cord that reduces the electrical flow, the information, from the brain to the body. When the bone or bones are adjusted into a better position to remove nerve pressure and cause less pain and proper function, as Dr. Jodon taught me, that is chiropractic.

As for my family, at the time of this writing, I have been married to the love of my life, Cassie, for almost 8 years. We are blessed with two beautiful and rambunctious sons, Cohen and Bennett, and are expecting our third in 5 months. My family is the most important thing in the world to me, so I do everything in my power to consistently show them how much I cherish them and what they mean to me. One of those ways, which to be quite frank is the most important, is to make sure they are healthy and keep them, and myself, steered on the Wellness Path.

CHILDREN AND THE WELLNESS PATH

Any parent would say that the number one priority in their daily lives is to ensure the safety and protection of their children. Most would consider this to mean physical and emotional harm, whether it be from bullies at school, images that they see on television, etc. Another one we want to look into is the priority of keeping our children as healthy as possible.

Remember the question a little earlier, "What of your body would you not want to function at 100%?" As a parent, an even more important question is asking what part of your child's body would you want functioning at less than 100%? Of course, that's a silly question. And honestly, have you ever thought of their health in that way? And if you have, or whether this is the first time you have contemplated it, what are you doing to ensure that? What CAN you do to ensure that? That, in essence, is the most important question to answer.

What we need to do is to discuss a few of the things that keep our kids from consistently being well. One of the most common issues parents see within their children is otitis media, more frequently know as your run-of-the-mill middle ear infection. Statistics reportedly show that 90% of all children will have contracted at least one ear infection while 20% of children will suffer from frequent ear infections[1]. A study done in 2015 showed 55% of children under one had suffered from an episode of acute otitis media[2]. Usually the course of treatment is antibiotics first. A meta-analysis of six studies was done in the late 90's that showed even though antibiotics could reduce pain in the 2-7 day range by 41% in the children who still experienced pain after day 1 (14%), antibiotics still only give a modest benefit[3]. They also concluded that antibiotics doubled the risk of vomiting, rashes, and diarrhea, as well as stating "to prevent one child from experiencing pain by 2-7 days after presentation, 17 children must be treated with antibiotics early." Those are not the greatest odds. Chiropractic research on the other hand, is very limited. A previous review showed 332 children being studied to see the outcome of chiropractic adjustments and ear infections. It showed that results were very favorable and there is a strong correlation to chiropractic and resolution to otitis media[4]. Within our office, we have seen cases of children suffering from ear infections in which we have also had very favorable results.

SICKNESS

Of course, what do kids seem to get very frequently, especially once they join a daycare of preschool? The sniffles. Whether that be from the common cold or allergies, when you child starts to come "under the weather," as a parent you start to get concerned. According to WebMD, preschool-aged children will average nine colds per year while kindergarteners will average twelve[5]! Does that seem like a lot to you? It certainly seems outrageous to me. And how is it usually treated. Cough syrups are used by 10% of American children every week[6], yet a study from 2009 shows that in the United States, and even Canada, they are not recommended for children under six due to the lack of evidence that they actually work and because of the health concerns associated with taking cough syrups[7]. Most do not know this. The real question though is why didn't anyone inform me of this? What's more, at the time of this writing, there is a study that's finally hitting the news cycle[8]. The University of Indiana concluded that very commonly used over-the-counter anticholinergic drugs increase the risk of decreased brain function, which can increase the likelihood of dementia[9]. And popular anticholinergic drugs used are Tylenol PM, Advil PM, Benadryl, Dimetapp, Dramamine, Paxil, and Unisom amongst others. What's sad and frustrating is that it seems the makers of these drugs have known this for many years. Yet the consumer, and the children of those consumers, are not finding out. Chiropractic adjustments have not been directly shown to decrease the time a cold takes to dissipate, however, it has been shown that 20 minutes after an adjustment there is a significant amount of immunoglobulin G synthesis evident, as well as synthesis of immunoglobulin M 2 hours after an adjustment[10]. And what are immunoglobulins, you may ask? The two that have been mentioned are released by the body when there is an infection present. You would want as much immunoglobulin present as needed for your children to fight off an infection, which in this case is the common cold.

As we have said earlier in this book, nothing within constitutes a doctor-patient relationship and all information not cited by research is individual opinion and do not ask or expect anyone reading to adopt a specific lifestyle. That being said, both of my young boys have been adjusted since a very early age. My first son was adjusted on day 5 and my second son was adjusted on day 3. They were not vaccinated when they were born, and still aren't. They did not get the erythromycin shot in their eyes or the vitamin K shot. My sons have both experienced fevers, but we have never given them Tylenol or any other chemical substance to reduce a fever. In fact most literature shows only when a temperature breaches 105°F does it becomes much more dire. The only antibiotics they have been given was for giving pink eye to each other.

OUR CHOICE

My family has made a choice; a choice we felt and feel is the best for our family. We do not like the side effects that come with the medications given for childhood issues. More importantly, we know that if they are fed nutrient dense foods and less sugar, they get sick much less often. From the moment they started getting regular food and drink, supplemented to them while my wife breastfed, they only drank water. My kids only ask for water when they are thirsty or when they are going to bed. We never had juice in the house because we knew that getting addicted to sugar can happen very early, reduce their immune system, and cause rapid tooth decay. My wife breastfed both of our boys until roughly 18 months old, which was around the time they both weaned themselves off to my wife's dismay. They get their spines regularly checked and adjusted and they get their vitamin supplementation. They are very healthy and ward off issues. I mentioned above the statistics on ear infections and colds. My older son turns six in a month, and my younger son is three years and four months old. They both have never had an ear infection and get one cold per year at most. We know that those outcomes are not an accident. We allow our boys' bodies to fight off and respond to external stimuli naturally. And yes, sometimes we supplement them with nonchemical means. On top of getting adjusted regularly and supplementing vitamins, another way we do our best to prevent issues in our children is to give them essential oils every evening on their feet.

In my opinion, the best way to help your children achieve a wellness lifestyle and guide them along a path of wellness is to model it and do it yourself. Children are smart little buggers; they pick up on things very quickly. And if they are talked to on a consistent basis on why you make the specific healthcare and lifestyle decisions you make for them, it will become more ingrained in them to live a healthy lifestyle themselves. A story I like to tell is when my family and I stayed in Estes Park a couple years back, my older son and I went to the grocery store. That night while I was there, I passed the bakery and all of a sudden was in the mood for a chocolate covered donut, yes, I am human. I went over to possibly grab one, and my older son, who was four at the time, scolded me and said, "No daddy, don't get that! It's not healthy for you!" Part of me was a little upset I wasn't getting a donut but more of me was very proud that he was understanding what the health environment was that he was being raised in, even at his young age, that your health is a CHOICE.

Each and every day, we have the responsibility as parents to make choices for ourselves and for our children. These choices that you make for them now will continue on even when they get older and become adults that get to make those decisions on their own. As parents, we are setting up our children's futures with the choices that we make for them and with them every single day. Give them the greatest gift you could possibly ever give them; the gift of optimal health. Their health at this point in their lives, if it starts to deteriorate or is lost for a period of time, it affects whether they are in school or not, but it also affects their relationships with other people, most importantly, the relationship with you, their parents. When your children are ill, who does that affect more, you or them? That's a very important question to ask yourself. And there is no better way that I can think of to ensure that kids are as healthy as possible than having a fully function nervous system free of spinal misalignments that can hinder their health. The means of doing that is gentle and specific chiropractic care.

REFERENCES

1. https://www.healthychildren.org/English/tips-tools/Symptom-Checker/Pages/symptomviewer.aspx?symptom=Ear+Infection+Questions
2. Nwokoye NN, Egwari LO, Olubi OO. Occurrence of otitis media in children and assessment of treatment options. J Laryngol Otol. 2015 Aug;129(8):779-83.
3. Del Mar CB, Paul PG. Are antibiotics indicated as initial treatment for children with acute otitis media? A meta-analysis. BMJ. 1997;314:1526.
4. Fallon J. The role of the chiropractic adjustments in the care and treatment of 332 children with otitis media. Journal of Clinical Chiropractic Pediatrics. 1997 Oct;2(2):167-183.
5. http://www.webmd.com/cold-and-flu/cold-guide/children_colds
6. Shefrin AE and Goldman RD. Use of over-the-counter and cold medications in children. Canadian Family Physician. 2009 Nov;55(11):1081-1083.
7. http://www.cnn.com/2007/HEALTH/10/19/coldmed.fda/index.html
8. http://www.cbsnews.com/news/popular-drugs-for-colds-allergies-

linked-to-dementia/
9. Risacher SL et. al. Association between anticholinergic medication use and cognition, brain metabolism, and brain atrophy in cognitively normal older adults. JAMA Neurol. Published online April 18, 2016.
10. Teodorczyk-Injeyan JA et al. Interleukin 2-regulated in vitro antibody production following a single spinal manipulative treatment in normal subjects. Chiropractic and Osteopathy. 2010 Sept;18(16):10.1186/1746-1340-18-26.

CHAPTER 7
TESTIMONIALS - OUR PATIENTS SPEAK

FROM KAREN A

"In August 2012, we made the decision that we were ready to start a family and decided to stop taking birth control and start trying. We didn't expect to get lucky on the first try but we also didn't expect that the journey would be as long and challenging as it was. A few months after stopping the pill, I began to have very irregular cycles. Sometimes they would be as short as 15 days and other times they would be upward of 100 days. After about 6 months of trying and several negative pregnancy test results, we sought out an ob/gyn doctor to find out what was "wrong" with me. The doctor talked to me about my weight (I was overweight but not obese, however I had gained approximately 30 lbs since first going on birth control in early 2010) as well as my diet and exercise. She did a lot of tests including a few ultra sounds to see if everything looked normal. For the most part everything was fine. The only thing she noted was that I was not producing maturing follicles when she thought I should be and she guessed that I might be missing my period every other cycle or so when I would have very long cycles. Since it had not yet been a year of trying, she suggested we take a break from trying and focus on losing at least 5% of my body weight. My husband

and I were really ready to start a family and so we decided that instead of working on preventing a pregnancy during this time of diet and exercise, we just wouldn't "actively try" (basically meaning that I wouldn't take my basal body temperature or test my cervical mucus each morning). While I was successful in losing some weight, my cycles never became normal and at one point the ob/gyn had to give me medication to make me re-start my cycle. At this point, the ob/gyn suggested that it was unlikely we would get pregnant on our own and suggested that we start Clomid. She also talked to us about IUI. She said that she would go through a maximum of 3 rounds with us and then if not successful, the next best idea was to start IVF. My husband and I left that appointment very upset and started talking about adoption. Neither one of us felt good about going through IUI or IVF... we wanted our baby made out of love for one another and didn't feel we could do that through IUI or IVF. We felt like, if we were supposed to have children naturally, then we would. Otherwise we would give a home to an unwanted child.

About this time, I attended a health fair through my work in mid-September 2013. I stopped by the Discover Health and Wellness booth and saw on their sign that seeing a chiropractor could help with infertility. I wasn't willing to ask the representative anything about this since my co-workers didn't know the challenges I was facing, so instead I signed up for one of their free sessions to meet the doctor. I met with Dr. Teets a couple weeks later and when he asked me about my health history, I brought up our challenges of conceiving a baby. He was the first doctor that we had seen that gave us hope to conceive naturally. He told me stories of others that he had helped and sent me to the DHW website to read about a case study. Even though we knew that we would struggle financially to see the chiropractor, my husband and I were impressed and hopeful, so we both decided to sign up for 6 months' worth of chiropractic care. We were hoping that if our bodies were aligned properly, that our bodies would "self-heal" and that my cycles would become normal.

As our care with Dr. Teets continued, he told us about a pill that he knew had helped others conceive. It is called Fertility Blend for Women and Fertility Blend of Men. After reading the reviews and talking to the ob/gyn, we decided that it didn't hurt to give it a try. We started taking the pills in late October 2013.

In mid-November we decided to purchase the Clearblue Fertility Monitor. I started testing (peeing on a strip and placing in fertility monitor to see my fertility level) on November 23rd, 2013. I received a peak fertility reading on December 13th and 14th and we did the baby dance!!! We spent Christmas in Baton Rouge, LA with family and returned to Denver Friday evening December 27th. As I made dinner, I sent my husband to the store to buy a test… I told him it would probably be negative but I just wanted to see…

I peed on the stick and before I could even lay it flat, I saw not one but 2 faint pink lines!!!! I started screaming for my husband and crying… I was so excited! I tested a couple more times that evening as well as the next morning and a few days after that and even a few more days after that. I couldn't believe that after what felt like a long challenging journey, that we were finally pregnant! The doctor finally confirmed our pregnancy at a 6 week ultra sound! We just made it to the third trimester and can't wait to welcome our little miracle to the world around September 4th!

We can't say for certain what allowed us to become pregnant. Was it the diet and exercise? Was it the Fertility Blend pills? Was it the chiropractic care? Was it understanding the timing through the use of the Clearblue Fertility Monitor? Or was it a combination of some or all of these things? Or was it just our time? We will never know. However, we do know that when we are ready to start trying for future children, that we will be using all of these methods again to hopefully conceive more quickly and avoid all the stress, tears, frustration, and depression that accompanies a diagnosis of infertility."

FROM LAUREN

"My name is Lauren and I heard about Dr. Wygonski and the office from my mom. When I first came in I had migraines really bad and I had a lot hip discomfort and shoulder discomfort. Since being under care the migraines have definitely stopped which is a drastic improvement. As far as my hip discomfort and shoulder discomfort it has reduced tremendously and I can do more exercises, I have more flexibility, and I am able to stand for longer periods of time. They're great people here and there's great care! They really care about whom you are and what's going on in your life. Not only just about your physical health but also what you're doing outside of that as well."

FROM GARY S

"Dr. Hanson, thank you for the follow up email. I wanted to say how much I appreciate you and thank you for working with me these past 6 months. You've been very patient, a great listener and so encouraging to me throughout my journey to better physical health. While the improvements are slow – they have been steady. I know that we are doing good things and that I will benefit now and for the rest of my life. One cannot put a price tag on that outcome."

FROM RON M

"I was referred to Discover Health and Wellness by a friend. She was in a lot of pain and found relief. When I first came in I had a number of things going on: neck pain, back pain, and I had just fractured my wrist. Since coming in for care I feel like I have better posture, I am in less pain, I feel stronger, and seem to be moving better. I like the fact that the doctor uses a non-invasive approach. I've been to a lot of chiropractors that do what I call "crack and rack" which can do a lot of damage. The way DHW approaches chiropractic is most effective for the least amount of trauma."

FROM P KEENS

"I am so thankful that I have met Dr. Zagiba and his staff! "Dr. Z" takes personal interest in each patient. He listens, provides guidance, and is your personal cheerleader; all this and he is great at what he does... spinal care / health and wellness. Three weeks ago I attended a class he provided on juicing. His passion and excitement motivated me so much that I have been juicing ever since. Dr. Z has also provided guidance on the type of yoga that is safest for my spine. I highly recommend Dr. Z and his staff at Discover Health and Wellness / Ken Caryl."

KIMBERLIN H

My husband DJ and I are both patients of Dr. Hall. DJ underwent a 6 month program to correct his neck issues and his results were amazing! The X rays Dr. Hall took at the beginning of treatment and after 6 months his neck was completely aligned. The weekly adjustments alone were not enough and Dr. Hall outlined various exercises DJ had to do nightly which took approximately 30 minutes. If you adhere to what Dr. Hall outlines and recommends you will benefit short and long term from the results. Not all chiropractors do X rays like Dr. Hall does. I feel it's a necessity for any reputable chiropractor to take them prior to setting up a protocol for a client. If you are in need of a chiropractor and live in Westminster or surrounding area definitely give their office a call.

FROM CARRIE M.

"We LOVE Discover Health and Wellness. Dr. Teets has put our whole family on a better path of health. Our 6 year old son has had years of chronic illness that none of Colorado's specialists could diagnose. And with DHW's chiropractic therapy, Avery finally got results. He is sleeping better, breathing better, eating better, and has had only one flare up on almost 8 months. We now have a little boy who can play and enjoy life like other kids! Thank you DHW! For years I have had headaches, pain down my neck and back, and pain and numbness in my arms. After my first 12 weeks, the pain was finally gone. I am feeling like new again. DHW has been a blessing for us all. Dr. Teets and his team have helped us learn how to think well, eat well, move well, and live well. Our experiences here have changed our lives significantly."

JERAMIE S

"About 18 months ago I moved about an hour out of town. I still make the trip down to Westminster to see Dr. Hall. I have Crohn's disease and digestive issues, and when I'm having a bad day, Dr. Hall knows exactly what to adjust and I walk out feeling like a new man. I've never met such a caring medical professional. I wish my General Doc was like this! He also is such a happy person, and it rubs off on you. When you go to see Dr. Hall you get an adjustment and a dose of positive energy. - Priceless."

FROM ANGIE

"My name is Angie, and I actually heard about Dr. Zagiba and Discover Health and Wellness from a team member at the Boat Show. I got a free chair massage and ended up coming in for a consultation. I've been coming maybe two and a half to three months now, and one of the things that I've noticed is that I'm in a health study for anxiety and depression and I have to take a monthly survey. And when I did my survey last month, it was the first time in the history of my life where I did not have any anxiety or depression symptoms. My anxiety and depression has pretty much gone away since coming and nothing else has changed in my life. This is the only thing that has changed is coming here."

FROM JOHN I

"I heard about Discover Health and Wellness from my niece, she was coming in for care and brought us in to get involved in the program. When I first came in I was very stressed and my shoulders were very stiff. I did not have the energy I thought I should have. Coming in for care has helped me with stress. I'm out of the mentality that when you're sick you need to go to the doctor, he will give you a pill, and you'll feel better. Whereas here, I feel like it's not just to relieve the pain in my back and shoulders, but it's to get my whole system going, give me energy, and to heal all my other problems that I'm having."

FROM ANGELA

"My name is Angela and I heard about Dr. Wygonski and Discover Health & Wellness through a health expo at my company. Prior to becoming a patient I had major aches and pains in my neck, upper, middle, and lower back which stemmed from bad posture due to a desk job for over 15 years. All of this contributed to me by not being about to sleep through the night because the pain was so discomforting.

My life has absolutely improved with regular weekly adjustment and exercises. I have noticed a decline in my back pain. I altered the way my work station is set up to include an ergo mouse and keyboard, a lumbar support added to my chair, and a foot rest to incorporate good posture. I have also decreased the use of over the counter medication on a daily bases. Chiropractic care works! I highly recommend coming to DHW to see how they can help you improve your quality of life."

FROM SARAH L

"We brought Leah to see Dr. Teets when she was 21 months old in hopes of dealing with recurring ear infections. After a winter with one ear infection after another, and one antibiotic after another, we talked to Dr. Teets about chiropractic adjustments and probiotics. Leah was also in speech therapy because her words were coming very slowly. Since Leah has been having adjustments and taking the probiotics (streptococcus salivarius K12) she hasn't had any ear infections! She has also had explosion of words and is no longer in speech therapy. We are so glad we tried chiropractic adjustments and probiotics instead of more antibiotics!"

FROM KRISTINE

"My name is Kristine and I heard about Dr. Wygonski and DHW through a friend who actually referred me when I was complaining about back pain. When I initially came in I had really bad pains in my lower back and my neck was always stiff and I was getting headaches a lot. Since I've been coming in, for about five months, I rarely have headaches and my lower back pain is essentially gone. Chiropractic does a lot more than I thought it would!"

FROM CYNTHIA R

"I discovered Discover Health and Wellness at a Pumpkin Chunkin Festival. I am a hair dresser and before coming to Dr. Hanson I had very stiff shoulders, chronic headaches and lots of fatigue. My life has improved since coming into the office. My headaches have completely disappeared, posture has improved, and I am managing my shoulder strain. There is an alternative to going to the doctor and just having medicine. It's a change of life style and one can be happy and fit!

FROM VIVIAN I

"I heard about Discover Health and Wellness from my niece. We've met Dr. Laszlo, and are very impressed with what he's doing here at Discover Health and Wellness. When I first came in I was pretty ill, I was fighting both a viral and a bacterial infection and was out of alignment and pretty much bed ridden. Through the massages, chiropractic and some nutritional advice, I am up and running and feeling pretty great. I think when I first started coming I was not a convert or a true believer right away. I was going through the motions of coming and showing up but then after each visit, or maybe a day or two later, I could tell I was getting stronger and stronger. I am able to keep up my activities now and do things I couldn't normally do. Before I couldn't cook a meal, I couldn't clean the house, and couldn't do my laundry. So this has really been a blessing to me. Chiropractic has come a long way in the last fifteen to twenty years, and I think that it's really good for the mind, body, and stress. The staff is very caring and goes out of the way to make sure you have the appointments that you need to get you feeling well. It's not just a number walking in, getting adjusted, and walking out. They care and become a part of your life."

FROM MELISSA S

"Dr. Zagiba is very knowledgeable and has a very genuine and personable approach with patients. His treatment plans are results oriented and his adjustments are always pleasant. I would highly recommend Discover Health and Wellness."

FROM KAREN S

"I am thrilled with Discover Health & Wellness! Dr. Hall is awesome and has helped me with so many of my hip, knee, and foot issues. I am so pleased with everything that I've experienced, I encouraged my husband to become a patient. Now we're both benefiting. Thank you!"

CONCLUSION

WELCOME AGAIN TO the wonderful world of wellness full circle! As we stated in the introduction, this book was written for the person who knows that our healthcare system isn't working. It was written for the person who knows that covering up the health of our body with more drugs and surgery is not how to stay healthy, vital, and energetic. This book is for the person that does not want the same health quality of life that their grandparents had. Discover Health and Wellness was written by caring, passionate Doctors of Chiropractic that are on purpose to change your life and to change the current broken model of healthcare as we know it. The Discover Health and Wellness purpose is to change the way our world views healthcare.

In summary, this book covered the aspects of what it means to Discover Health and Wellness. Wellness is a combination of understanding the importance of our bodies own innate intelligence. It is about seeing how important nutrition is to your overall wellbeing. Wellness is about unlocking the keys to looking good and feeling good through exercise and fitness. Wellness is about having the mindset to be empowered and in control of our wellness warrior. We went in depth explaining how your nervous system works and the importance of wellness care for our children. Lastly, our patients shared their stories on how their lives have been transformed by Discover Health and Wellness and their new found approach to healthcare.

As you have gone through these chapters, we feel confident that you have been armed with the tools to take control of your health, to no longer be dependent on the current model of sick care. This book was meant to empower you with rejuvenating health freedom. Don't be a statistic. The Leading Causes of Death and Disability in the United States such as heart disease, stroke, cancer, type 2 diabetes, obesity, and arthritis—are among the most common, costly, and preventable of all health problems. *Center of Disease Control Feb 23, 2016*

Through a healthy posture and nervous system, nutrition, and exercise, our Discover Health and Wellness protocols help prevent the majority of preventable diseases!

THE PROBLEM

Our current model of healthcare is expensive, it doesn't work very well, and it's dangerous. It is very expensive. It is bankrupting our nation. It doesn't work! Our current model of taking medication for symptoms is making us sicker and sicker. Medicine is dangerous! It causes over 750,000 deaths a year. That's as many as heart disease and cancer.

A study in the Journal of the American Medical Association stated that the US has the most expensive system, by far. It also stated that the US Healthcare system is a dysfunctional mess. *JAMA May 16th, 2007* The New England Journal of Medicine stated that the American healthcare system is at once the most expensive and the most inadequate system in the developed world. *NEJM Jan. 7th, 1999* It is evident that the American Medical System is the leading cause of death in the United States. The total number of deaths is 783,936. *JAMA Barbara Starfield, MD 2000* The British Medical Journal stated that, medical errors now kill an estimated 250,000 Americans a year." *BMJ 2016* Something fundamentally is going wrong to cause our country to lose ground against other high income countries." *NIH and NAS 2013*

THE SOLUTION

We are affordable, have a better model of healthcare, and we are extremely safe. We have the Solution! We're the answer that you've been looking for. We have affordable care plans. If you committed to your care plan, we are committed to making a plan work for you. We have a better model of healthcare. Many times medicine is vital and necessary. The problem is that we have mistaken medicine for health care instead of crisis care. We teach our patients how to take care of themselves proactively and naturally so they don't need medicine. It is all about natural first/drugs last – It is about getting to the source of the problem not covering up symptoms. We are extremely safe.

Leading US researchers conducted the largest study of its kind of chiropractic care. They found a strong connection between those receiving chiropractic care and self reported improvement in health, wellness, and quality of life. 95% of participants said their expectations had been met. They reported making better food choices, took less medications, got sick less often, had more energy, and had far less symptoms. Journal of Vertebral Subluxation Research 1997;1(4):15 Another study stated that persons receiving chiropractic care reported better overall health, spent fewer days in hospitals and nursing homes, used fewer prescription drugs, and were more active. *Topics in Clinical Chiropractic 1996;3(2):46.* Lastly, another study showed that chiropractic patients receiving maintenance care spent 31% less than the national average for health care services and experienced 50% fewer medial provider visits. Journal of Manipulative and Physiological Therapeutics 2000;23(1):10. We are the answer.

OUR PURPOSE

Our Discover Health and Wellness team believes that each and every one of us are here for a purpose. Our purpose is to change the way the world views healthcare. By empowering you with this health freedom and this choice for wellness, we believe we are able to help you achieve your purpose by feeling your best!

We want to leave you with what we believe to be fundamental to living the Discover Health and Wellness lifestyle. Once you are feeling your best, we believe life is most magnificently experienced by three main drivers to happiness: Gratitude, Potential, and Service.

Let's start with gratitude. Wake up every morning in a state of gratefulness. Be grateful for the day. Be grateful for everything in your life. You were created to shine. There is only one you and you were beautifully and wonderfully made. There's a plan for your life. Continue to believe deep down to your soul, that you were made for a reason. I believe that we must first know ourselves, discover what we are good at, discover what makes us feel alive, and then go do what we were gifted to do. So number one, be grateful. You'll be happier inside and you'll develop a sense of peace and understanding that surpasses everything.

Secondly, be your best. The main recipe I know of for emotional disaster is to not become what you know you are capable of. Whatever you can be, you must be. Believe in yourself. You can be what you want to be. Break those shackles of inhibition and go after what you want. Aren't you happiest when you're growing, accomplishing something, going after what is important to you? If you fall down, get back up. Keep moving forward. You are worth it. Be your best.

Lastly, help others. Contribute. I don't believe we were born to keep our talents to ourselves. I believe we have a moral right to help others and bring them closer to their purpose, to give them opportunities to elevate themselves. Don't you feel great when you are helping someone with your time or money? Have you done that lately? Who needs help around you? Who do you know that truly wants to better themselves? Help someone today , small or big, give it a shot. Help others.

On behalf of the entire Discover Health and Wellness team, thank you for empowering your health. Good things are going to happen. God bless and keep smiling.

ABOUT THE AUTHORS

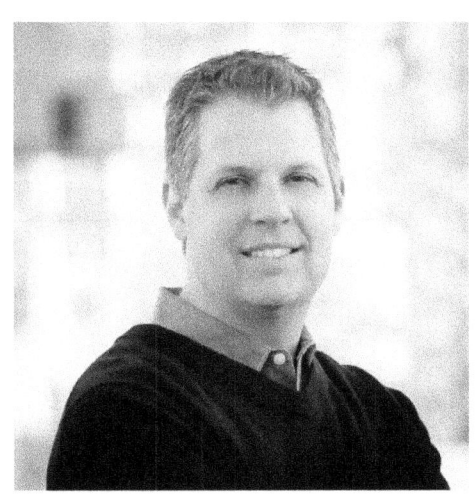

DR. KEPPEN LASZLO – FOUNDER AND EXECUTIVE DIRECTOR

DISCOVER HEALTH AND WELLNESS

A passionate advocate for health, Dr. Keppen Laszlo is the Founder and Executive Director of Discover Health and Wellness. Setting out to change the landscape of healthcare by delivering patient-centered, results-driven chiropractic care, Dr. Laszlo opened the first Discover Health and Wellness office in 1999. The Colorado community embraced this approach, and today Discover Health and Wellness is one of the largest health and wellness centers in the state.

Dr. Laszlo also developed the non-profit organization, The Elevate Foundation, which is dedicated to the education of health and wellness across the United States.

He is the best-selling author of the book Elevate – The Ultimate Life Success Formula and a contributor to the NY Times best-selling book, Body by God and One Minute Wellness. He has been a featured speaker at Barnes and Nobles and a frequent guest on NBC's Colorado and Company.

Dr. Laszlo is an award winning presenter and has shared the stage with the likes of: Mark Randall, Mike Koenigs, Bill Phillips, and John Assaraf. And although he has given the message of Elevate all over the country, he still has the duty of cleaning up the coughed up cat hairballs at home.

He resides in Broomfield and loves spending his time with his beautiful wife, their two fabulous boys, and is on purpose to inspire greatness through courage, potential and fulfillment.

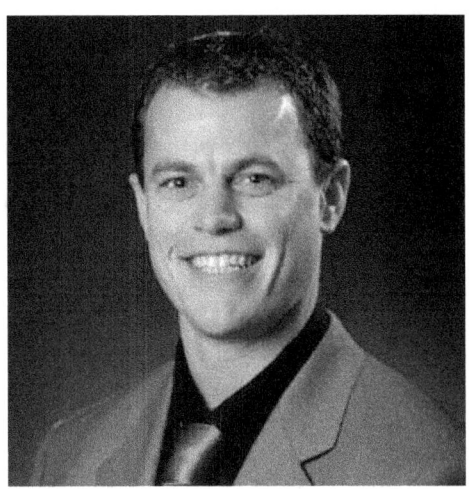

DR. ANDREW HANSON – DOCTOR OF CHIROPRACTIC

DISCOVER HEALTH AND WELLNESS, DENVER

"It is my life's passion, my pleasure and my mission to give Denver residents the chiropractic care they need and deserve. I want to share my and DHW's vision to offer healthy healthcare with the communities of Cherry Creek, Glendale, Aurora and surrounding communities.Our purpose at DHW is to change the way our world views healthcare. It's my goal to do this every day by educating all our patients how to properly take care of their spine while dealing with stress and toxicity. Additionally, I hope to inspire my patients to become the best person they can be by staying pain-free and keeping the body balanced so that the nervous system can function properly.

"I grew up in Pierre, South Dakota ,where I excelled in Football, Basketball and Tennis. As the quarterback of my high school team, I developed a passion to lead that has remained with me throughout my life. I started my college career in South Dakota where I graduated from a Civil Engineering program. In 2004, I decided to take a risk and move away from my family and friends to attend Colorado State University. At CSU, I received my Bachelors in Sports Medicine and also fell in love with Colorado and the mountains.

"After a life changing illness and personal victory in my own health with chiropractic care, I developed a passion for chiropractic and what it had to offer to the world. As a result, I have since dedicated my life to sharing the powerful message of chiropractic. In 2008, I attended Parker University in Dallas, Texas and graduated in December of 2011with my Doctorate of Chiropractic. Following graduation, I did a short postceptorship, where I learned from some great chiropractors and furthered my understanding of the miraculous human body. In May of 2013, I joined the wonderful doctors and staff of Discover Health and Wellness and went on to open our beautiful Denver location.

"I am always expanding my education and knowledge by attending seminars and education classes yearly. If a challenging case comes into the clinic, I can tap into over 43 years of combined experience by consulting with one of the other doctors at DHW. In my free time I enjoy every aspect of Colorado by hiking, trail running, snowboarding, golfing, Crossfit training along with a host of other outdoor actives. I am one of five siblings and I'm very close to my parents, sibling and many nieces and nephews. I welcome you to join DHW's family of patients. May this year be the year you discover the best version of you."

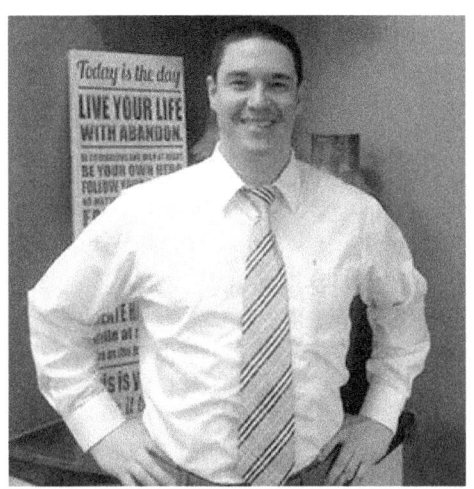

DR. CAMERON HALL – DOCTOR OF CHIROPRACTIC

DISCOVER HEALTH AND WELLNESS, WESTMINSTER

"I am originally from West Virginia so I am a mountain boy. I grew up in the ski industry and that is where I first encountered chiropractic. As a Senior Ski Patroller, I was on my skies for up to 10 hours a day. We had a chiropractor there on staff and without his help and treatment, I would have been retired much earlier from skiing. After my first adjustment with my knees I went from being able to spend only 2-3 hours on the slopes to a full 8-hour shift. It was amazing. My original degree is in genetics, but it wasn't long before I found out that I wasn't cut out for microscopes and small sterile rooms.

"My path eventually lead me to chiropractic and I haven't looked back since. What turned me on to the path of chiropractic was the different point of view Doctors of Chiropractic have. We look at the body as a single functioning unit. Your body is an amazing machine and if something is altered in its structure there will be far-reaching side effects. Not only pain, but altered biomechanics which can cause joint degeneration and arthritis.

"By looking at your bodies biomechanics, Doctors of Chiropractic can identify areas that will be prone to injury, degeneration and early arthritis. Correcting altered biomechanics will help to prevent these issues. Doctors of Chiropractic can also identify areas of your nervous system that are under stress and pressure. Any alteration in your bodies boney alignment will cause pressure to be applied to the nervous system. Over time this pressure can lead to nerve damage and decreased function of whatever those impinged nerves innervate. Realigning the proper bony segments will relieve that pressure and allow those nerves to function properly.

"This is why I chose to become a Doctor of Chiropractic. To work with your body in a safe, effective, and efficient method of treatment that not only prevents future medical issues but also gives you real time benefits. I chose Colorado because I love the mountains and I love to ski. Chiropractic allows me to pursue my passions and to also keep my own body at its peak performance so I can enjoy my passions like they were meant to be."

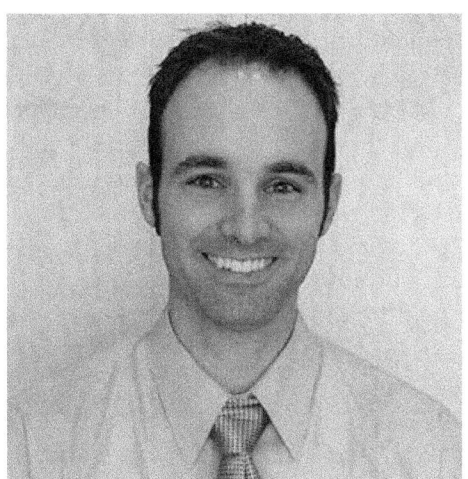

DR. BRANDEN TEETS – DOCTOR OF CHIROPRACTIC

DISCOVER HEALTH AND WELLNESS, LONE TREE

"When I was 16 years old, my life changed. I was an all-county cross-country runner, but one day during a training run a had a back spasm so intense it made me drop to all fours and took me out of that day's workout. A friend on the team told me to see his dad, a chiropractor, and that "he would fix me." I didn't even know what a chiropractor was, in fact, I had never heard the word before. But if it meant I could run again, I was willing to do anything. So after seeing him for about 2 weeks, my back issues were gone and could run again with no issue.

"That wasn't all. Something more profound happened about five weeks into care. I noticed, all of a sudden, a slew of gastrointestinal issues that I had dealt with since childhood disappeared! I told him about it, and he informed me of what chiropractic was all about. It wasn't about how "he would fix me." It was centered around how I fixed myself; he was only there to put my spine into better alignment so that my body could do what it was made to do, which is heal itself and thrive.

"My passion for natural health care has only intensified as the years have added on. There are too many suffering people out that that don't know how detrimental spinal misalignments are for their current and future health. Too many people are drugging symptoms, and gaining more symptoms from those drugs, instead of finding the source of a problem and eliminating it by allowing the body to heal itself. That is why I decided to pursue a career in chiropractic care. After I earned my undergraduate degree in Biology from Saint Vincent College, I went to receive my Doctor of Chiropractic degree from Live University in Marietta, Georgia. As for other passions, they are first and foremost my wife, Cassie, and two boys, Cohen and Bennett. I love to run and have been doing so since age 13. I have run races from 5Ks to a marathon. My current fitness goal is to qualify for the 2017 Boston Marathon."

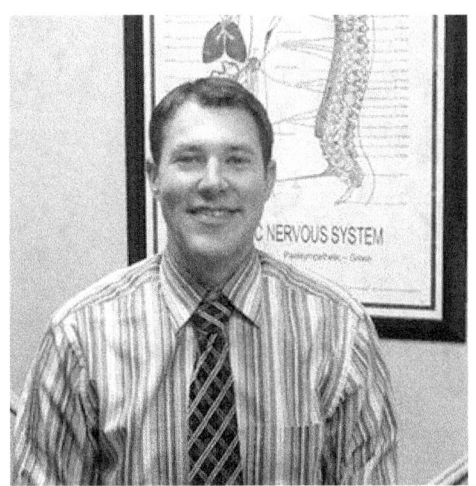

DR. PHILLIP WYGONSKI – DOCTOR OF CHIROPRACTIC

DISCOVER HEALTH AND WELLNESS, NORTHGLENN

"I got into this profession because there is no better doctor then the one inside each of us. I believe symptoms are an expression of your body trying to tell us that something is not right. Most people weren't born with their symptoms but they developed over time. I look to find the source and correct it if possible or refer out though our network of healthcare professionals. I promise to not waste your valuable time if you are looking for answers.

"On days when I am not in the office I am spending time with my wife. We enjoy being active in the outdoors. We enjoy skiing during the winter months and mountain biking in the summer months. We also just bought our first house that is a fixer upper. All those HGTV shows made restoring a house look easier than it is."

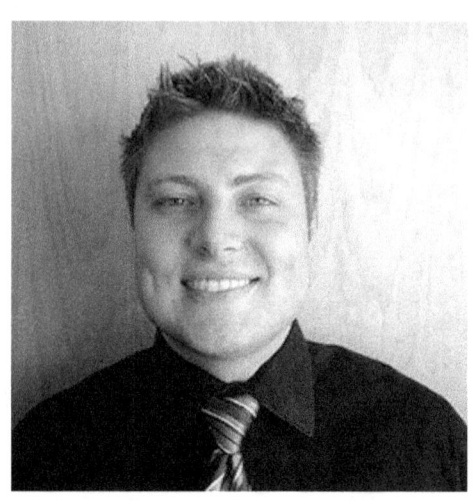

DR. DALE ZAGIBA – DOCTOR OF CHIROPRACTIC

DISCOVER HEALTH AND WELLNESS, KEN CARYL

"I am originally from New Jersey, but spent most of my childhood in North Carolina. I was inspired at a young age to become a doctor. My uncle was paralyzed from a neck injury sustained in a pool diving accident, this began my fascination for spine and healthcare. After the passing of my mother, and strong support from my father, I decided to begin my journey to become a Chiropractor. I just knew there had to be a better way to approach health.

"After excelling in athletics and academics in high school, I pursued my undergraduate degree in exercise physiology from East Carolina University. After graduating with honors, I then proceeded to earn my Doctor of Chiropractic from Palmer College of Chiropractic Florida campus. There I learned how I could use Chiropractic and a health minded lifestyle, to take a more proactive model to health.

"I enjoy practicing at Discover Health and Wellness Ken Caryl, and living in colorful Colorado with my wife, Lindsie, and our son Anthony.

"At Discover Health and Wellness I get to take my knowledge and skills, and use my passion for helping people change their life through improving their health. I just want everyone to know that I care about you and I am there to give you the same quality care I give my family."

www.ingramcontent.com/pod-product-compliance
Lightning Source LLC
Chambersburg PA
CBHW060155290526
45789CB00003B/1048